Trigger Poin Therapy with Foam Roller and Massage Ball:

Exercise Manual for Self Myofacial and Deep Tissue Massage to Stop Your Muscle and Joint Pain

Legal & Disclaimer

The information contained in this book and its contents is not designed to replace or take the place of any form of medical or professional advice; and is not meant to replace the need for independent medical, financial, legal or other professional advice or services, as may be required. The content and information in this book has been provided for educational and entertainment purposes only.

The content and information contained in this book has been compiled from sources deemed reliable, and it is accurate to the best of the Author's knowledge, information and belief. However, the Author cannot guarantee its accuracy and validity and cannot be held liable for any errors and/or omissions. Further, changes are periodically made to this book as and when needed. Where appropriate and/or necessary, you must consult a professional (including but not limited to your doctor, attorney, financial advisor or such other professional advisor) before using any of the suggested remedies, techniques, or information in this book.

Upon using the contents and information contained in this book, you agree to hold harmless the Author from and against any damages, costs, and expenses, including any legal fees potentially resulting from the application of any of the information provided by this book. This disclaimer applies to any loss, damages or injury caused by the use and application, whether directly or indirectly, of any advice or information presented, whether for breach of contract, tort, negligence, personal injury, criminal intent, or under any other cause of action.

You agree to accept all risks of using the information presented inside this book.

You agree that by continuing to read this book, where appropriate and/or necessary, you shall consult a professional (including but not limited to your doctor, attorney, or financial advisor or such other advisor as needed) before using any of the suggested remedies, techniques, or information in this book.

Table of Contents

Trigger Poin Therapy with Foam Roller and Massage Ball: 1

Exercise Manual for Self Myofacial and Deep Tissue Massage to Stop Your Muscle and Joint Pain 1

Introduction 5

Chapter 1: Benefits Of Using Foam Roller 6

    1. Increased Mobility 6

    2. Pain Therapy 7

    3. Improved Functions Of Our Vital Organs 7

    4. Improved Vitality 8

    5. Reduction Of Cellulite 8

Chapter 2: Different Types Of Massage Rollers 10

    1. Soft Body Roller 11

    2. Rumble Roller 11

    3. Textured Foam Roller 12

    4. Cold Foam Roller 12

    5. Textured Ball Roller 13

    6. Foot Roller 13

    7. Adjustable Foam Roller 14

    8. Wand Foam Roller 14

Chapter 3: Foam Rolling Safety Tips 15

Chapter 4: The Exercises 18

    1. Inner Thigh (Adductor) 18

    How to Do Inner Thigh Foam Rolling 18

    2. Biceps Release 18

    How to Do Foam Rolling For Biceps Release 19

    3. Total Calf Release 19

    How to Do Total Calf Release Foam Rolling 19

    4. Hamstring Release 20

    How to Do Hamstring Release 20

    5. Lower Back (Erector Spinae) 21

    How to Do Foam Rolling for Lower Back 21

    6. Piriformis (Upper Buttocks) 22

    How to Foam Roll for Piriformis 22

7.   Glute Massage 22

How to Do Glute Massage 23

8.   Sacrum Release 23

How to Do Sacrum Release 23

9.   Upper Back (Rhomboids) 24

How to perform the Upper Back Foam Rolling 24

Chapter 5: Lacrosse Ball and Spiky Ball Workouts 25

Lacrosse Ball Exercises 25

1.   Glutes Massage 25

2.   Hamstrings Massage 25

3.   Upper Shoulders And Back 26

4.   Foot Massage 26

Common Spiky Ball Exercises 27

1.   Shoulder Release 27

2.   Gluteal Release 27

3.   Foot Release 28

Conclusion 29

Introduction

A foam roller is a cylindrical log that is used as workout equipment for its usability and convenience. It was in fact initially used as a tooling aid during physical therapy sessions but has become an important part of a good workout regimen. It is a terrific product for self-massage, core stability, balance training, regular stretching, pain management, yoga exercises and Pilates.

An individual might occasionally suffer from muscle pains because of the tightening up of the tissues. This tightening of the muscle tissue is usually known as muscle knot or simply a trigger point. To ease pains linked to the trigger points, one has to diffuse somehow or break up the knots. The roller is a type of exercise equipment that stretches muscular tissues and tendons plus it breaks down scar tissue formation and soft tissue adhesions. Using your very own body mass on the cylindrical foam, you'll be able to conduct a self-massage, reduce trigger points and ease tight fascia. The pressure of the body on the foam will even enhance blood flow and circulation to your soft tissues. A foam roller is an effective tool that can help in preventing injuries, managing pain, and self-myofascial release. Much like the gymnastic rings, rollers may also be utilized for balance training.

They come in one-foot and three-foot long cylindrical sizes and are also manufactured from top quality hard foam. Whenever getting a foam roller, be sure to check out its feel, firmness, and thickness. There should be no huge holes or perforations as it may cause it to be lumpy, making this useless. You could get a great massage on the IT (iliotibial) band with a foam roller. Just lie on the ground on your side and roll backward and forwards over the roller in between the knee and hip. For the lower leg, move backward and forwards from above the ankle to your knee. Together with IT bands, you can also do massage on your huge muscles in the legs like quads, calves, and hamstring, middle back stretching.

In doing any exercise, ensure that you comply with some specific key points so that it is going to be effective and worthwhile. You need to devote a minimum of one minute rolling forwards and backward on the hurting or tight muscle areas. Refrain from rolling over the bony areas of the body. It is recommended to work with a roller for 5 to 10 minutes just before doing exercises.

The goal is to massage those areas to release pressure and lessen muscle density. Remember, however, that you'll encounter pain while utilizing the roller, primarily on the first few days of usage. As you utilize it often, you are going to work through the tightness and temporary soreness.

Chapter 1: Benefits Of Using Foam Roller

Foam rolling has many more benefits than most people are aware of. It goes way beyond simply soothing tired and sore muscles (though this is one of the major benefits), to so many peripheral health benefits, it might amaze you. In this chapter we will briefly cover some of the benefits you can expect to achieve from a regular foam rolling routine. It is really quite hard (if not impossible) to list all of the benefits you can expect to achieve, as there are quite literally too many benefits to count. Not only are there so many benefits of foam rolling that several books could be written on just the benefits alone, but science and health care professionals are finding new benefits just about every day.

Once you've finished reading this chapter, you will understand why foam rolling is one of the most helpful workouts you can do for your body. You will find that foam rolling is a natural holistic approach to keeping yourself healthy, improving your life drastically, and staving off many effects that come with aging. You will realize that foam rolling may be the most important, life-changing, a decision you have ever made.

1. Increased Mobility

One of the effects of aging seems to be a decrease in many people's mobility. That is to say, activities that were once easy and pain-free become more difficult as we age. We may find that simply walking, bending and reaching become strenuous and (for some) even impossible. Many people are convinced this is just a normal process of aging and that there is really nothing we can do about. I have even heard some doctors tell their patients that their decreased mobility is simply them "getting older" and it is part of life.

Most physical therapists, especially those who specialize in geriatric therapy, will agree that the main cause of limited mobility in the elderly is due to joint inflammation and muscular degradation, as well as gross myofascial adhesions throughout the body. As we will discover in this chapter, one of the main benefits of foam rolling is an increase in the blood flow throughout the body. Much older and older adults may have poor circulation which causes the joints and ligaments to stiffen up, due to improper lubrication and a decreased nutrient-rich blood supply.

The good news is that foam rolling isn't limited to young, healthy, vibrant individuals, but that anyone, from 3 years old (perhaps younger) to 90 years old (perhaps even older) can benefit from foam rolling.

It is especially a very useful addition to any rehabilitation program, in that it can be applied as gently or firmly as necessary, to massage and loosen adhesions and improve circulation throughout the body.

2. Pain Therapy

One of the main benefits of foam rolling is in easing the pain in tired and sore muscles, but the pain therapy of foam rolling goes way beyond this. Not only is foam rolling highly beneficial to joint and muscle therapy, but it can also help ease or erase pains that often go untreated for years, or are treated with pain medications that only cover the symptoms and never actually treat them.

First, your muscles, tendons, ligaments and joints are constantly being pulled, stretched, and often misused in ways that gradually break them down and cause them to "malfunction." Arthritis, bursitis, tendonitis and a host of other conditions occur with the misuse and mistreatment of muscles over a prolonged period, causing pain in our later years and often limiting our mobility. By practicing effective foam rolling techniques (which are presented later in this book), you can stave off these conditions and possibly even reverse some of these conditions.

A daily foam rolling regimen, especially in the upper back and shoulders, can provide a very deep and wonderful release to these nerves, by smoothing out the muscle and tissue and allowing you proper balance of your head/neck. Many people have expressed surprise at how much foam rolling has relieved their headaches, but headaches are not the only aches, and pains foam rolling has been shown to relieve.

3. Improved Functions Of Our Vital Organs

Not only does increasing the blood circulation (by breaking up fascial adhesions) decrease and often eliminate much pain, but our organs begin to operate at peak performance, doing the jobs at which they are best. I don't have to tell you how important it is that your heart continues to pump blood throughout your body, or how important it is for your kidneys to continue to eliminate waste products from the blood and control the water fluid levels.

By releasing fascial adhesions through foam rolling, you will improve that blood circulation, ensuring that these vital organs get the proper amount of oxygen and nutrients so that they can continue to function. Many people have told me that, while they expected that their mobility would be improved and possibly some aches and pains would be alleviated, they were quite pleasantly surprised (and often shocked) by how much better they felt overall after adhering to a regular foam rolling regimen. These are benefits of foam rolling directly related to the improvement of vital organs.

4. Improved Vitality

As your vital organs receive the proper flow of blood, your energy levels will naturally increase, due to your body finally working the way it is supposed to. A healthy circulation is of utmost importance to our overall health and vitality.

One of the comments that I have heard from every single person who has decided to take up foam rolling and have stuck to a regime for a couple of weeks is that they were surprised how energetic they had become. Many have told me that they have been sleeping much better, often sleeping fewer hours and feeling even more refreshed than ever before.

The great thing about this new level of vitality is that you can use it to get your body into even better shape. You now have the energy (and ambition) to exercise regularly, increasing your strength and endurance. You may find that walking is not only easier now, but even more enjoyable. Your blood oxygen level will go up even more through activities you may have avoided, and as this happens your vitality will increase even more. In other words, you will find that simply starting a regular rolling regimen may drastically increase your quality of life in ways you couldn't even imagine.

5. Reduction Of Cellulite

In case you don't know, cellulite is a condition that causes the skin to appear to have areas of underlying fat deposits, which gives the skin a dimpled, lumpy appearance. It is most often noted on the thighs, abdomen, and buttocks. There are many different medical terms used to define cellulite, such as adiposis edema tosa, dermopanniculosis deformans or status protrusus cutis. You don't need to know the medical terminology to recognize cellulite, which is also often called orange peel syndrome or cottage cheese skin (which is much more descriptive than the medical terms).

While you could plop down a hundred dollars for some miracle cream that might (or might not) help you to reduce your cellulite, but will more than likely leave you worse off, you will find that foam rolling does the job quite nicely and not only does it help reduce (or completely eliminate) this excessive cellulite, but it will keep it off indefinitely as long as you continue to roll.

Foam rolling has been shown to massage those areas and help to break up the interwoven fat fibers that may contribute to cellulite build up. Rolling also increases the flow of blood (and oxygen) to those areas which in turn help to keep the underlying fibers healthy and functional as well as helping your body to eliminate fluids and toxins. If you are like thousands of others with cellulite in your thighs, abdomen or buttocks, within a few short weeks of foam rolling, you will notice that this cellulite seems to simply melt away, without any additional supplements or dangerous creams.

Foam rolling benefits us by allowing us to break up many adhesions that are causing our body to struggle to provide nutrients and oxygen to all of our organs, and many serious conditions can be found rooted in this poor circulation.

Not only is our circulation improved and our vital organs receive the oxygen and nutrients they need, but the muscles, tendons, and joints are improved, increasing our mobility which increases the number of healthy activities we can comfortably participate in.

I can go on for days telling you about all of the benefits I have heard from clients and friends who have given foam rolling a try, but I think the best way to understand these benefits is to experience them for yourself. Foam rollers are not expensive, can be stored easily and are pretty fun to use, once you get the hang of them.

Therefore foam rolling, while requiring daily adherence, is an activity you will enjoy, looking forward to doing it daily.

Chapter 2: Different Types Of Massage Rollers

Foam rolling is a way that can be used efficiently to work out many muscles including the TFL, trapezius, rhomboids, hip flexors, hamstrings, quadriceps, adductors, piriformis, latissimus forsi and gastrocnemius. By rolling these muscles over the foam roller with maintained amount of pressure, these muscle groups can be relaxed and eased. Now it's time to talk about the equipment used in this self-massage technique.

Foam rolling is recommended either for warming up or recovering. As part of your warm up exercise, foam rolling prepares you for the intense workout you need to do. It will improve your blood flow. With blood properly circulating, it reduces your risk of injuries. After a workout, foam rolling also comes highly recommended. It can help speed up your muscle's recovery time because it further improves your blood flow and thereby bring much-needed nutrients and oxygen to your muscles.

The foam roller is typically in the form of a cylinder. It comes in many sizes, but the most commonly used is around 6 inches in diameter and about 12 inches in length. The long foam rollers, however, can measure up to 36 inches long. The longer rollers are typically used for the back. Since you are a newbie to foam rolling, it is best to start with the softer kind. To help you get acquainted though, I will be introducing you to the different shapes and sizes of foam rollers.

Before anything else, you should know that there are two major kinds of foam rollers:

1. The EVA foam roller
2. The EVE high-density foam roller.

EVA rollers are especially soft. Now, this may be favorable if you want a soft touch. And it may be good for you as a beginner. The downside is it flattens easily. You're lucky if you can make EVA foam rollers last a year.

The EVE foam roller, on the other hand, offers a much firmer touch. It may not be as soft as EVA rollers but EVE's can withstand the abuse. They can last for several years.

How do you tell them apart? You can judge a roller by its color. EVA rollers usually are white while EVE high-density rollers usually come in darker colors. Most of them are black. Moreover, EVA rollers have a smooth texture. EVE rollers, on the other hand, are more textured. They may look like they have small pellets on the surface.

So you better watch out! Mind your choice.

1. Soft Body Roller

This type of foam roller is recommended for beginners although non-beginners also use it. The soft body roller is for anyone who favors the soft kind of touch. You can massage your major muscle groups using this cushy roller. This is ideal for the thighs and the back.

Beginners start with foam rollers that are of a larger diameter. If the foam roller's surface is bigger, then foam rolling becomes more tolerable. That's because the pressure is dispersed rather than concentrated. Once you are ready to increase the intensity, you can start switching to the smaller diameter kind.

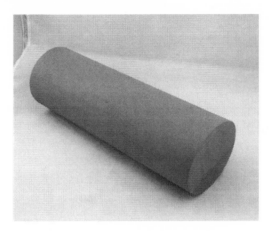

2. Rumble Roller

This is reserved for people who long for intense touch. If you want to go deeper, this foam roller is for you. However, if your pain tolerance is low, you better steer clear from this roller.

Notice that this foam roller has bumps. You can use them to release super-tough knots. Avoid using this roller for too long in one area unless you want to hurt yourself even more and cause more damage to your muscles.

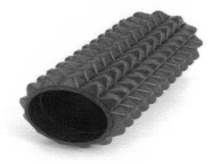

3. Textured Foam Roller

This is an all-purpose foam roller. Get this equipment if the soft roller's too soft but the hard roller is too intense for you. It will give you a little more intensity. You can get a little more pressure with this one.

This foam roller is designed with grooves and bumps. This kind of design allows you to zero in on tight areas. You can roll back and forth on tight spots. With the textured foam roller though, you can pause on that specific spot. Work on contracting and relaxing the muscle as you rest on the roller. The grooves and bumps will do the work for you.

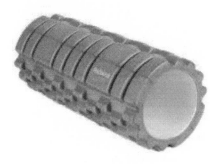

4. Cold Foam Roller

If you are looking for a cool relief, this may be the right roller for you. It can do wonders for nagging injuries and intense aches.

The cold foam roller is made of stainless steel. If you are feeling sore after your workout, roll this cold ball over your sore muscles. It can provide instant relief, and it's preferable than an ice bath. The cold foam roller offers quicker recovery time and lesser risk of inflammation.

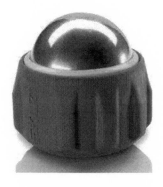

5. Textured Ball Roller

So you don't like intense pressure, but you do have some sore spots you need to work on. This foam roller is for you.

The orbs in this roller can be used to target smaller muscle groups including those in your hips. It is best for a much-targeted pressure. As a matter of fact, you can adjust the firmness of the roller according to how tight the muscle feels. You can make the necessary adjustments using a needle inflating pump.

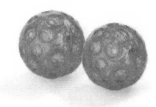

6. Foot Roller

This is good for people who suffer from tired feet, especially those of runners. This special roller is designed to help with tight soles. Use it under your calves or feet. The foot roller can be used for small areas. It is made of dense knobs that feel like the fingertips of a massage therapist.

Avoid rolling directly to the tightest muscle. It won't be as effective as you hope it will be. That's because the tightest muscle will be restricted. It will be much harder to get it to relax. If the muscle is not relaxed as you roll, the massage won't result in anything.

You may even want to work on your lower legs first. Roll your way down to your feet. Or you can begin by rolling on your back and hips with a lacrosse ball. You can then move the ball to your torso before you start using the foot roller from your legs to your tight soles.

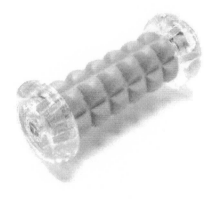

7. Adjustable Foam Roller

This adjustable roller is truly a knot buster. It is specially designed to work out the knots and kinks on your calves, hamstrings, and quads.

Instead of resting your body over the roller, you can hold onto the roller's ergonomic handles and roll it over your target spot. You can simply push the bar against the spot in an upward and downward motion. The contoured roller will make sure the muscle group is properly treated. The disks on this roller will rotate as you push up and down to release the knots. You control the handle which means you can push as gently or as firmly as you please.

If it gets too intense rolling on your troubled spot, you can try deep breathing. It will help with the pain.

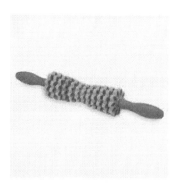

8. Wand Foam Roller

Runners may benefit most from this wand foam roller. This is a variation of the adjustable roller with handle. The wand is designed with a strip of foam which can be rolled slowly over your IT band, calves, hamstrings and quads. Do not rush the process. Roll as slowly as you can so that the fascia can loosen up. The effectiveness of your rolling session depends on this.

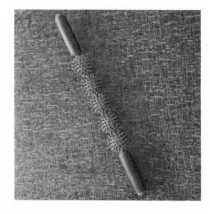

Chapter 3: Foam Rolling Safety Tips

Foam rolling used to be an exclusive practice among professional athletes, coaches, and physical therapists. It has now become a widespread practice. Because of its benefits to health, foam rolling is practiced by individuals from various levels of fitness.

Most of them started where you are, clueless and a bit confused. To help you in the process, I've laid out here some basic foam rolling guidelines. Follow them correctly, and you are sure to reap the many benefits of this Self-Myofascial Release technique.

1. **Stretch first-** You must be eager to get started. Before you do, stretch on the area you will be working on first. Do stretch before you roll on that muscle group. It doesn't even have to be an elaborate one as long as it is properly warmed up.

2. **Position your body properly-** The foam roller should be under your body. The body area should rest directly on the foam roller.

3. **Expect discomfort-** As we mentioned previously, a little pain or discomfort is expected. If you're rolling on a trigger point, the pain may radiate in other areas of the body as well. This is normal.

4. **Apply gentle pressure-** The idea here is to use your body weight in that specific area to apply pressure. Start slowly and stop only at the level you can tolerate. Roll on the target area back and forth.

5. **Keep rolling until the discomfort subsides-** Your main focus should be in tight areas. These areas can be especially painful. Work on inflexible areas too. Foam rolling will help regulate normal blood circulation. It will not only fix the knots. It will also help improve muscle flexibility.

6. **Do not roll on joints and bones-** Roll on muscles and soft tissue. Avoid rolling directly over your joints and bones. Foam rolling won't do anything for these hard parts except unnecessary pain.

7. **Do not roll too quickly-** To properly work on the muscles, you need to roll slowly. Rolling fast in a back-and-forth motion is not advisable. In fact, you should not exceed an inch per second.

Rolling faster may hurt less but to truly treat the knots, you need to apply slow and deliberate movements. This is how you can achieve the main goal which is to relax the muscles and release the fascia. Releasing the fascia cannot be rushed. After all, the fascia is composed of fibrous and thick web of tissue. Going it over in a quick pass simply won't work.

8. **Do not stay in the same spot for too long-** Foam rolling is not a test of endurance. It's not about how long you can handle it. Rolling on one spot for too long will do more damage. You run the risk of damaging the tissue or irritating a nerve. This may not only lead to bruising. It may, in fact, worsen the inflammation which is the last thing you want.

9. **Do not roll directly on the injured area-** If the area is too painful to even without rolling, it could only mean one thing. The area is injured. Avoid constantly rolling on it as it may only lead to further tension and make the inflammation worse. Focus on the connecting tissue. Do it slowly and apply pressure gradually.

10. **Mind your form and posture- to** maximize the results of foam rolling; you need to follow the correct form and posture. Otherwise, you may only do more harm than good. If you find yourself too tired to foam roll, take your time to rest. It is important that you are properly focused throughout the entire foam rolling session.

11. **Do not roll on your lower back-** It is okay to roll the upper back, but it is best to avoid foam rolling the lower back. Using a foam roller for this body part will make the spine contract as a protective effort. If you are experiencing pain from your lower back, you may use a lacrosse or tennis ball instead. Or better yet, consult a professional about the best way to deal with such a problem.

12. **Wait for 1 to 2 days before another session-** It is not advisable to perform foam rolling sessions every other day. Although you need to do this regularly, you still have to wait it out around 24 to 48 hours before the next session. In the meantime, stay hydrated. Keep in mind that trigger points may also be caused by other lifestyle factors including nutrition. Make healthy improvements on your diet. Make sure you are well rested.

13. **Consult with your doctor first-** Foam rolling is beneficial. However, it may not be recommended for all. People suffering from skin conditions, bleeding disorders, kidney, heart, and organ failure may steer clear from this technique unless their doctor has cleared them. Always check with your doctor. A health professional can provide further advice on proper use of the technique so you can maximize its benefits.

Finally, keep these guidelines in mind when performing foam rolling exercises.

Chapter 4: The Exercises

1. Inner Thigh (Adductor)

Inner thigh foam rolling is the best workout for tight thighs, since you will be able to open them up. Yu will definitely like this foam roller exercise to a deep massage. By foam rolling the full round foam roller over your inner thigh, you will loosen tough connective tissue and minimize stiffness in your muscles.

How to Do Inner Thigh Foam Rolling

- Place yourself into a plank stance on your toes and elbows.
- Lay your full round foam roller at an angle of 45° to your body.
- Gently open your left knee out, while rotating your foot at your hip.
- Lay your left inner on the full round foam roller jus over the knee.
- Slowly roll the roller from your knee towards your inner thigh.
- Keep a good amount of weight as you can.
- Repeat the whole process with the opposite leg.

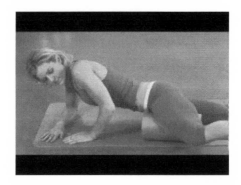

2. Biceps Release

Body muscles are known to move in pairs; well, when the biceps are the leading overs, and they contract to bend the arm. On the other hand, the triceps respond as the release. While the triceps contract, the biceps release, and your arm will straighten out. You should know that when a single muscle group is not balanced on the opposing group; then tension may increase. Therefore, it is important to engage foam rolling for biceps release.

How to Do Foam Rolling For Biceps Release

- Lie down while facing down with your right arm extended to the side and your left arm in a comfortable position to provide support.
- Place the full round foam roller at the top of your right biceps.
- Apply tender pressure into the foam roller.
- Hold on the current position for a few seconds.
- The roll your body gently to roll the foam roller along your biceps.
- Apply static pressure as required to deal with any tight spots, and hold for as long as possible.
- Make certain to breathe slowly and fully.
- Repeat the whole process for the opposite arm.

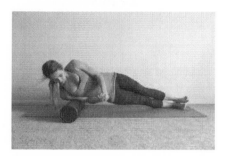

3. Total Calf Release

Of all the muscle groups in the human body, the calves are the most affected by genetics. Ideally, they can be the most challenging muscle group to develop. Nevertheless, you can always improve the size and condition of your calves. A feature unique to calves is that they can be exercised with more regularity than other muscles. An ideal workout for managing healthy calves is total calf release.

How to Do Total Calf Release Foam Rolling

- Sit on the floor with your legs are straightened out, and your hands positioned behind your supporting your weight.
- Place a full round foam roller under your knees.
- Slowly roll along the back of your legs side by side from your knees to your ankles.
- Continue rolling to locate a tender spot, and then apply adequate pressure.

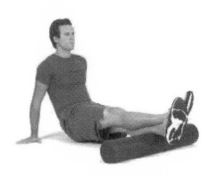

4. Hamstring Release

Hamstring release is best employed to minimize hamstring hyper-tonicity. This exercise employs the norm of counter-strain to treat dysfunction between agonist and antagonist muscle groups. Root goal of hamstring release includes but is not limited to: improving sitting balance and posture; minimizing internal rotation in gait; improving stride length; decreasing abnormal pull that can cause hip dislocation; decreasing compensatory ankle; and eliminating inefficient crouched gait pattern.

How to Do Hamstring Release

- Sit with your right leg position on a full round foam roller.
- Bend your left knee, and place your hands on the floor behind you for support.
- Roll up and down from your knee to just under your right butt cheek.
- Switch legs and repeat the whole process.

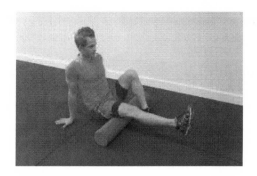

5. Lower Back (Erector Spinae)

Foam rolling on your lower back helps to stretch the abdominal as well as lower back muscles. The exercise also trains the pelvis in a neuromuscular manner as you move from one position to another. The focus of this exercise is to isolate middle back movement. However, this particular workout is not appropriate for people suffering from injuries as well as the unstable lumbar spine.

How to Do Foam Rolling for Lower Back

- Lie on the floor while facing up, and place a full round foam roller across your back, just below the point of your shoulder blades.
- Place your hands behind your neck for support.
- Arch your back over the foam roller while keeping your hips and lower back on the mat.
- Hold at the current position for a few seconds, relax, and then repeat the stretch for a couple of times.

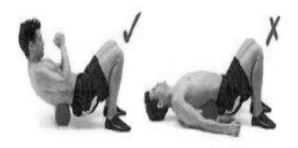

6. Piriformis (Upper Buttocks)

Piriformis is situated in the gluteal area and helps to rotate the thigh externally. The Piriformis are a highly essential group of muscles that be flexible and have improved balance. This drill is quite easy to do, and the resulting outcomes are very beneficial to the general body health and movement.

How to Foam Roll for Piriformis

- Start in a seated position on a full round foam roller, while your right leg crossed over your left knee.
- Use your right arm to support your weight by placing it on the floor behind you.
- Gently roll the foam roller across the exterior of your hip, just above the gluteal area.
- Switch legs and supporting position and repeat the whole process.

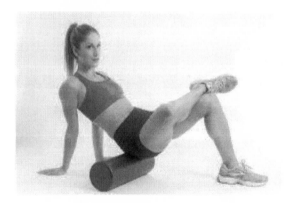

7. Glute Massage

Glute Massage using foam rollers releases locked glutes from sitting. The release of glutes effectively increases blood flow to the hip musculature and reduces glute-induced back strain, and it mobilizes hips as well as the low back. However, you are supposed to avoid this exercise if you experience a sharp pain or if you are in the acute phase of sciatica. Furthermore, you need to maintain a small range of motion if you have had a hip replacement.

How to Do Glute Massage

- Gently position yourself on the floor with a full round foam roller just under your bottom.
- Roll side by side along your Glute for at least thirty seconds.
- Check for tender spots while rolling, maintain the roller at a tender spot in case you locate one for a few seconds.

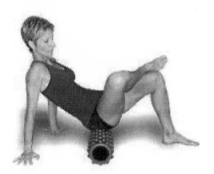

8. Sacrum Release

The sacrum consists of five vertebrae bones attached into the shape of a triangle that has a gentle posterior curve. The sacrum top vertebral bone forms a joint with the fifth lumbar vertebra. The lowest vertebral bone forms a joint with the tailbone.

How to Do Sacrum Release

- Lie on your back, place a soft full round foam roller under your sacrum.
- Slowly roll side by side on the roller, while exploring for a position that gives comfortable pressure into the sacrum.
- Remember that comfort is your guide; therefore, find the angles of zero pain.
- Allow yourself at least three minutes for this exercise.

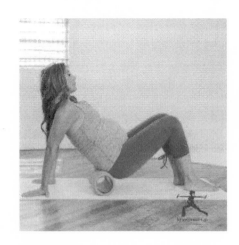

9. Upper Back (Rhomboids)

The upper back muscles (Rhomboids) attach to several vertebrae of the upper back as well as to the interior edge of the shoulder blades. The function of the Rhomboids is to move the shoulder blade toward the spine, to help raise the shoulder blade and to hold the shoulder blade still when needed. This acts as a solid support for the functioning of the arm and the hand. Trigger points in the upper back refer pain along the inner edge of the shoulder blade. Massage can be applied easily and efficiently using a foam roller.

How to perform the Upper Back Foam Rolling

- Lie face up with a foam roller under your upper back that is at the bottom of your shoulder blade
- Bend your knees at a 90-degree angle with your feet flat on the floor
- Hold your hands behind your head and pull your elbows towards each other pointed to the sky
- Slightly raise your hips off the floor
- Lower your head and upper back slowly, and roll from your shoulders down to the middle of your back
- Repeat the performance by raising back to the start and hold your position on sore spots for an extended time

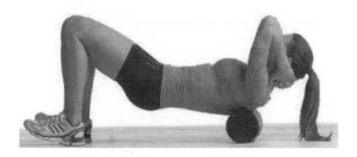

Chapter 5: Lacrosse Ball and Spiky Ball Workouts

Lacrosse Ball Exercises

1. **Glutes Massage**

- Stand with your back upon a wall with the lacrosse ball.
- Sway side to side and up and down until you find a soft spot.
- Allowing the ball to apply pressure on this area, relax your weight into the wall.
- Until you feel the pain subside hold this for 30 seconds.
- Repeat on another side.

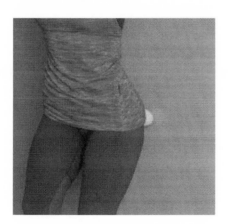

2. **Hamstrings Massage**

- Sit on a hard chair that's high enough off the ground to let your legs hang.

- Put the lacrosse ball beneath your thigh, and moving it until you find a soft spot.
- Slowly bend and extend your knee for 30 seconds.

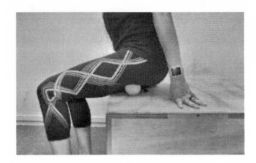

3. Upper Shoulders And Back

- With a lacrosse ball between your upper back and the wall stand with your back against a wall.
- Place the ball on one side of your spine.
- Move around in all directions until you find a soft spot.

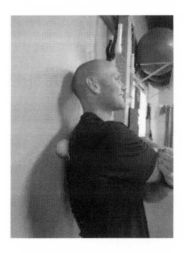

4. Foot Massage

- With your feet on the floor relax comfortably.
- Under the arch of your foot put the lacrosse ball.
- Slowly move the ball along the arch of your foot.

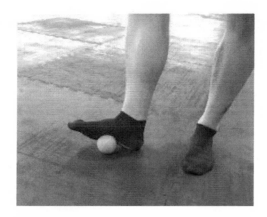

Common Spiky Ball Exercises

1. Shoulder Release

- Standing with your Spiky Ball on the wall
- Applying pressure to any areas which feel tight apply your body weight to move the ball.

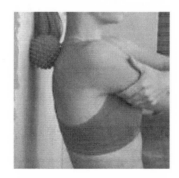

2. Gluteal Release

- Lie on your back with your feet flat on the ground and knees bent.
- Put your Spiky Ball underneath your buttocks.
- Smoothly roll over the ball until you find a trigger point.
- To increase the pressure, let the knee on the affected side drop out to the side.

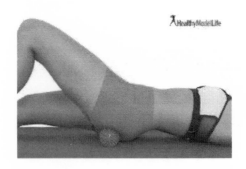

3. Foot Release

- Place the Spiky Ball underneath your foot.
- Apply your body weight to the foot to roll the ball from your heel towards your toes.

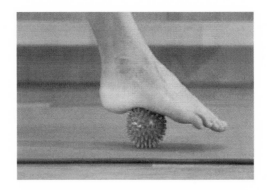

Conclusion

If you've made it all the way through this book, congratulations!

You've learned how foam rolling came about, what exactly self-myofascial release is about and why foam rolling can help you in keeping yourself limber with full-range of motions in your joints and muscles.

You've also learned that by utilizing your foam roller daily, you can add years to take years or your life off your life (as in feeling younger), by increasing your circulation and keeping your muscles from knotting up.

As you progress in your rolling exercises, you may even find yourself improvising and coming up with new techniques. Just remember, when you do any self-myofascial release, there should be very little pain and no strain on any muscles.

So save your money, save your muscles and save your mobility, get yourself a foam roller and get to feeling better, more energized and healthier through self-myofascial release.

Made in the USA
Middletown, DE
12 September 2018